COLOUR GUIDE

Hand Conditions

Douglas W. Lamb MB ChB FRCS(Ed)

Formerly Consultant Orthopaedic Surgeon and Surgeon in Charge of Hand
Clinics at the Royal Infirmary, Western General Hospital and Princess Margaret
Rose Orthopaedic Hospital, Edinburgh; Honorary Senior Lecturer in
Orthopaedic Surgery, University of Edinburgh; Past President of the
International Federation of Societies for Surgery of the Hand

Geoffrey Hooper MMSc FRCS(Eng) FRCS(Ed)(Orth)

Consultant Orthopaedic Surgeon, Princess Margaret Rose Orthopaedic Hospital
and the Royal Infirmary, Edinburgh; Honorary Senior Lecturer in Orthopaedic
Surgery, University of Edinburgh

Churchill Livingstone

EDINBURGH LONDON MADRID MELBOURNE NEW YORK AND TOKYO 1994

CHURCHILL LIVINGSTONE
Medical Division of Longman Group UK Limited

Distributed in the United States of America by
Churchill Livingstone Inc., 650 Avenue of the Americas,
New York, N.Y. 10011, and by associated companies,
branches and representatives throughout the world.

© Longman Group UK Limited 1994

First published as Colour Aids—Hand Conditions 1985

ISBN 0 443 04972-6

British Library Cataloguing in Publication Data
A catalogue record for this book is available from the
British Library.

Library of Congress Cataloging in Publication Data
A catalogue record for this book is available from the
Library of Congress.

Publisher
Michael Parkinson

Project Editor
Jim Killgore

Editor
Adele Mighton

Production
Nancy Arnott

Designer
Design Resources Unit

Sales Promotion Executive
Marion Pollock

The
publisher's
policy is to use
**paper manufactured
from sustainable forests**

Printed in Hong Kong
GC/01

Acknowledgements

We wish to thank the following for generously providing illustrations: Department of Orthopaedic Surgery, University of Edinburgh (Figs 43, 90); Department of Dermatology, University of Edinburgh (Figs 91, 135); Mr R. Bryson (Figs 52, 102); Dr E. Housley (Figs 53, 131, 132, 133); Dr K. Little (Figs 81, 82).

We thank Michael Devlin and Sonia Miller for their help in the preparation of photographic material and Alison McGowan for her assistance with the manuscript.

Edinburgh   D. W. L
1994   G. H.

Contents

1 / Complications of injury

Swelling

Swelling of the hand (Fig. 1) is the result of crushing injuries, dependency and immobility. A protein-rich fluid fills the tissue planes and, if not dispersed, will encourage the moving parts of the hand to adhere, with disastrous loss of function. After any injury or elective surgical procedure swelling must be minimized or prevented by keeping the hand elevated and starting active movement as soon as possible. Carefully supervised physiotherapy has a major role in the care of hand injuries.

Dangers of sling
Swelling of the hand will diminish considerably after even a few hours of elevation. The traditional broad arm sling is useless and often dangerous in hand injuries for it may allow the hand to adopt a dependent posture and cause constriction of the wrist at the edge of the sling, both of which will increase swelling.

Correct elevation
If the hand is swollen it should be elevated in a roller towel or similar proprietary support (Fig. 2). This will require hospital admission but will almost certainly prevent a prolonged and possibly permanent period of disability.

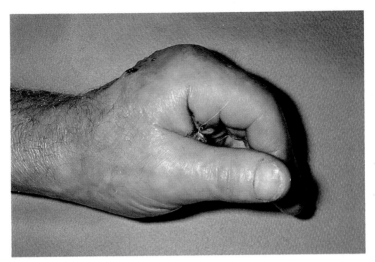

Fig. 1 Swelling of the hand after injury.

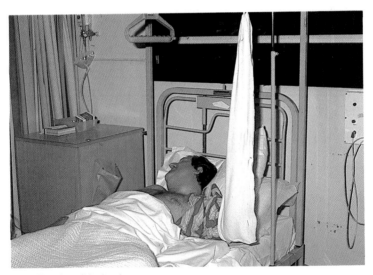

Fig. 2 Elevation of the hand.

Contractures

Improper splinting of the injured hand will cause contractures of the collateral ligaments of the small joints in the hand (Fig. 3) and may convert a minor injury into a permanent disability. Incorrect splintage must be avoided (p. 9).

Position of splintage

If the hand must be splinted it is important to keep the ligamentous structures of the joints of the digits at their full length to prevent contractures. The ligaments are fully stretched when the interphalangeal joints are straight and metacarpophalangeal joints flexed to 90° or, in the case of the thumb, when it is fully abducted from the palm (Fig. 4).

Method of splintage

Boxing glove: this position can be maintained by a 'boxing glove' dressing (Fig. 5) in which the fingers are splinted round a pad of fluffed gauze in the palm by wool and crepe bandages. The wrist must be kept dorsiflexed and this is best done by reinforcing the dressing with a plaster back slab, which also holds the bandages in place.

Volar slab: as an alternative to the boxing glove dressing the hand may be placed in a volar slab in the position shown in Figure 4.

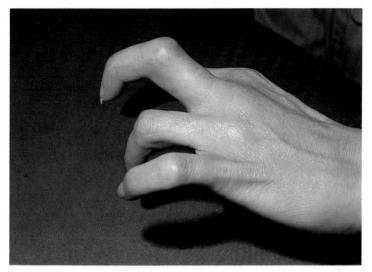

Fig. 3 Fixed flexion deformity of the long finger.

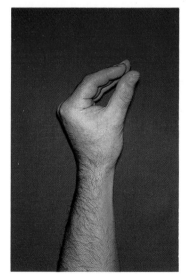

Fig. 4 The correct position for immobilization.

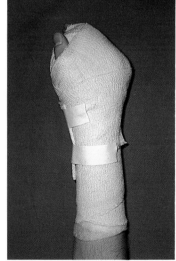

Fig. 5 A boxing glove dressing.

Reflex sympathetic dystrophy (RSD)

Definition & clinical features
A condition of unknown cause that may follow minor injuries or surgical procedures on the hand. It is characterized by severe pain, stiffness and vasomotor changes in the skin (Fig. 6). In the established case patchy osteoporosis is seen on the radiograph (Fig. 7).

Synonyms
Sudeck's osteodystrophy; algodystrophy.

Prevention
Established RSD is difficult to treat but the condition can be prevented by encouraging movement of the hand as soon as possible after injury.

Volkmann's contracture

Definition
Ischaemic fibrosis of the forearm muscles that most commonly occurs after a supracondylar fracture of the humerus in childhood.

Pathology
Impairment of the microcirculation by raised pressure in the fascial compartments containing the muscles. If not treated urgently permanent muscle damage and secondary fibrosis will occur.

Clinical features
Severe and increasing pain aggravated by passive extension of the fingers. Later fibrosis of muscles and ischaemic damage to nerves produces a claw hand and flexion of the wrist (Fig. 8).

Management
Early: release tight bandages and gently extend the elbow; if no response the deep fascia should be released surgically.
Late: splintage and reconstructive surgery may improve function.

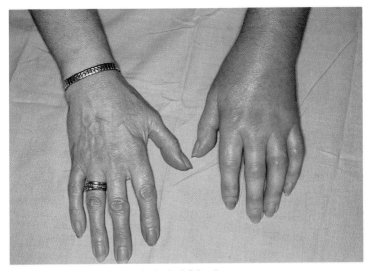

Fig. 6 Reflex sympathetic dystrophy in the left hand.

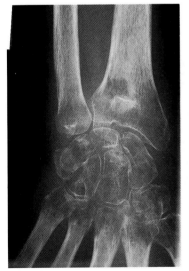

Fig. 7 Patchy osteoporosis in established RSD.

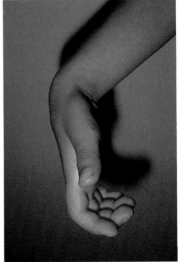

Fig. 8 Volkmann's ischaemic contracture.

2 / **Fractures**

Phalangeal fractures

Undisplaced Undisplaced, stable fractures of the phalanges (Fig. 9) do not need elaborate treatment. Healing is rapid and movement of the finger should be encouraged as soon as pain and swelling allow.

Displaced Displaced fractures (Fig. 10) should be reduced and held on a splint (p. 9) for 2–3 weeks. When the fracture is clinically stable supervised mobilization is started.

Although the majority of phalangeal fractures can be treated by conservative methods, if a fracture is unstable and continues to displace when splinted it may be necessary to stabilize the fracture by internal fixation. Malunited fractures, especially of the proximal phalanx, produce an unsightly deformity of the finger (Fig. 11).

Intra-articular Fractures that enter the joint, for example condylar fractures (Fig. 12), often require internal fixation with fine Kirschner wires or screws to control reduction and allow early mobilization.

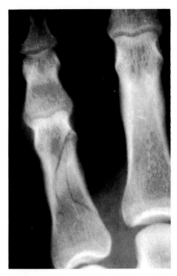

Fig. 9 A stable undisplaced fracture of the proximal phalanx.

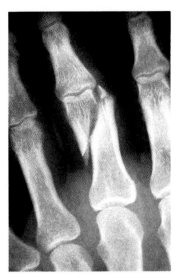

Fig. 10 An unstable displaced fracture of the proximal phalanx.

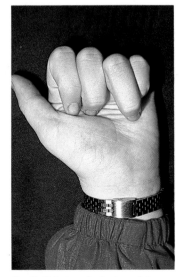

Fig. 11 Malunion of a fracture of the proximal phalanx of the ring finger.

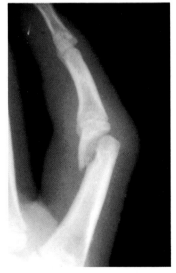

Fig. 12 A condylar fracture of the proximal phalanx.

Phalangeal fractures (contd)

Treatment by splintage
The type of splintage used depends on the displacement and instability of the fracture.

Type of fracture

Stable fractures: these are treated by splinting the injured finger to the adjacent one using garter strapping (Fig. 13) or a similar proprietary splint. The joints should be free to move and it is important to have protective padding between the fingers to prevent pressure sores over bony points.

Displaced fractures: displaced phalangeal fractures can be held after reduction on a metal splint padded with foam rubber (Fig. 14). The right–angle bend in the splint should be placed at the metacarpophalangeal joint, the surface marking of which is the distal palmar skin crease.

Complications
To avoid malrotation when using a metal splint, the palmar part of the splint should point to the tuberosity of the scaphoid which is the point to which the fingertips converge when the fingers are flexed. Malrotation of the finger on the splint can be checked by looking at the fingernails from the tips of the fingers. Normally the nails of all four fingers make segments of a smooth arc which is broken when one finger is out of alignment.

The finger should never be splinted straight on a tongue spatula (Fig. 15) or flexed over a roller bandage (Fig. 16) because secondary joint contractures are very likely to occur when these methods are used (p. 3).

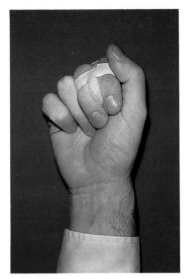

Fig. 13 Garter strapping.

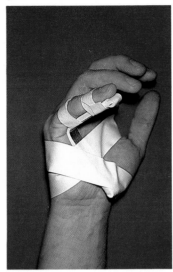

Fig. 14 The use of a padded metal splint.

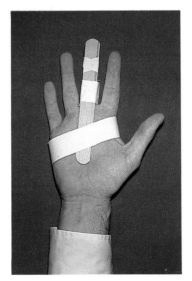

Fig. 15 Incorrect splintage of metacarpophalangeal joint in extension.

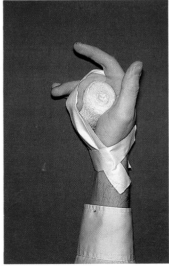

Fig. 16 Incorrect splintage of interphalangeal joints in flexion.

Metacarpal fractures

Isolated fractures of the metacarpal shafts are usually stable and, as they are splinted by adjacent bones, additional splintage is unnecessary. Displaced fractures may need reduction and stabilization.

Boxer's fracture

A fracture through the neck of the little finger metacarpal bone (Figs 17 and 18) is extremely common. It is usually caused by striking an object with the ungloved fist.

Management Splintage is not necessary and early active mobilization should be encouraged. The loss of prominence of the knuckle is not a problem as it does not interfere with hand function. Reduction and internal fixation is only indicated in the uncommon case in which there is marked displacement of the metacarpal head.

Bennett's fracture

A fracture–dislocation of the base of the thumb metacarpal bone (Fig. 19). The small fragment remains in the correct position while the first ray is pulled proximally by attached muscles.

Management Redisplacement is common after reduction and it is advisable to stabilize the first ray in the reduced position by a Kirschner wire driven into the trapezium or adjacent metacarpal bone. The wire is removed some 4 weeks later when the fracture has healed.

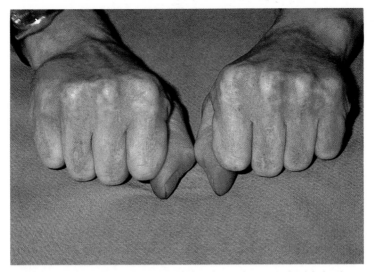

Fig. 17 Loss of prominence of the knuckle after a boxer's fracture in the right hand.

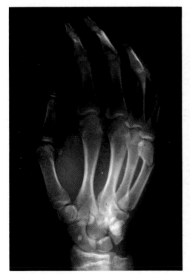

Fig. 18 Boxer's fracture.

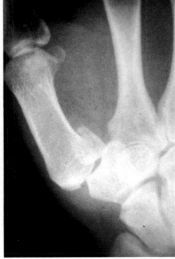

Fig. 19 Bennett's fracture.

3 / Carpal injuries

Fracture of the scaphoid

The scaphoid is usually broken (Fig. 20) in a fall on the outstretched hand. It is a common injury in young men.

Clinical features The wrist is painful and there is tenderness in the 'anatomical snuff–box' at the base of the thumb.

Management If a fracture of the scaphoid is suspected but not seen on X-ray examination it is wise to splint the wrist and arrange for a further examination in about 10 days. Most fractures will unite after splintage for 8 weeks in a forearm cast but delayed or nonunion are indications for surgical treatment by bone–grafting and internal fixation. Established nonunions (Fig. 21) are often discovered when a patient develops pain in a wrist that was 'badly sprained' some years before.

Dislocated lunate

This injury (Fig. 22) is one of a group of carpal dislocations that share a similar mechanism of injury. They are associated with disruption of the ligaments of the wrist and intercarpal instability may persist after reduction.

Kienböck's disease

Avascular necrosis of the lunate (Fig. 23) is thought to be triggered by minor trauma. It usually affects young people, causing pain in the wrist. Osteoarthritic changes may develop in the longer term.

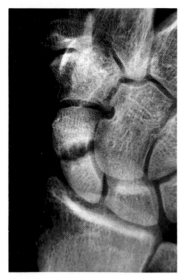

Fig. 20 Scaphoid fracture.

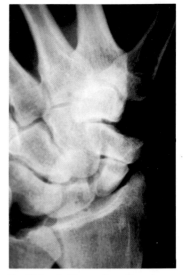

Fig. 21 Scaphoid nonunion with early osteoarthritic changes.

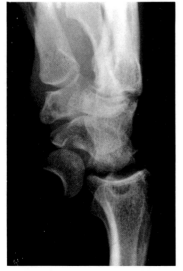

Fig. 22 Dislocation of the lunate. Lateral view.

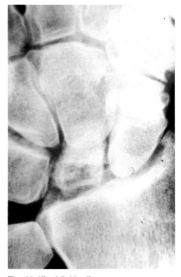

Fig. 23 Kienböck's disease.

4 / Joint injuries

Dislocations

Dislocations most frequently occur in proximal interphalangeal joints. The intermediate phalanx may be dislocated dorsally (Fig. 24), laterally or, more rarely, anteriorly.

Management Even though the dislocation is usually obvious on clinical examination an X-ray examination should be done before and after reduction to exclude associated fractures and check congruity of reduction.

Reduction is straightforward and can be carried out with ring–block anaesthesia. Damage to the collateral ligaments should be checked by stressing them after reduction (Fig. 25). Surgical repair may be needed if a ligament is torn.

Unless there is a torn ligament the joint is splinted for a few days until acute pain has subsided.

Complications Ligamentous injuries of the proximal interphalangeal joints, whether or not the joint has been dislocated, are often followed by prolonged swelling (Fig. 26) and discomfort — 'spindle finger'. Patients should be warned that this may occur as they are often reluctant to move the joint when it is swollen.

Stiffness and flexion contractures can rapidly become established in the proximal interphalangeal joint after injury, but can be prevented by correct splintage and early mobilization as soon as the acute discomfort is resolving.

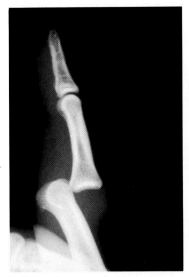

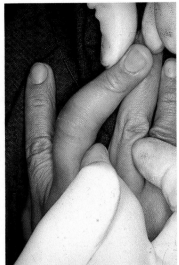

Fig. 24 Dorsal dislocation of the proximal interphalangeal joint.

Fig. 25 Rupture of a collateral ligament.

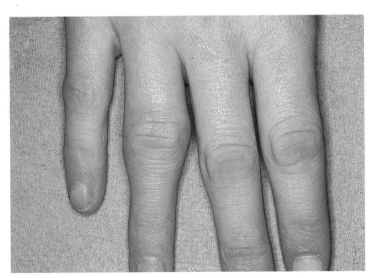

Fig. 26 Swelling of the proximal interphalangeal joint after a minor sprain.

Ulnar collateral ligament injury in the thumb

Sprains and ruptures of the ulnar collateral ligament of the metacarpophalangeal joint of the thumb are common injuries.

Mechanism This injury is caused by an acute abduction strain applied to the thumb, often during sporting activities such as skiing. Chronic stretching related to occupation may occur ('gamekeeper's thumb').

Diagnosis Rupture of the ligament should be confirmed by stressing the joint after injecting local anaesthetic into the tender area (Fig. 27). A radiograph taken when stress is applied will show subluxation of the joint (Fig. 28). Occasionally a fragment of bone is avulsed from the proximal phalanx (Fig. 29) with the ulnar collateral ligament.

Management An acute sprain should be treated by a cast that includes the thumb for 3–4 weeks. If the ligament has ruptured completely this is not an effective form of treatment because healing is prevented by the adductor aponeurosis which becomes interposed between the ligament and base of the proximal phalanx of the thumb. Operative repair of the ligament is necessary to prevent chronic instability of the thumb.

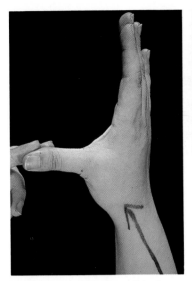

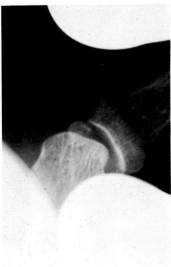

Fig. 27 Rupture of the ulnar collateral ligament of the metacarpophalangeal joint of the thumb.

Fig. 28 Subluxation of the joint on a stress view.

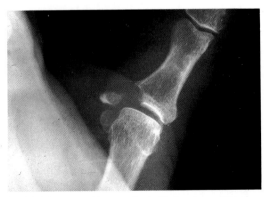

Fig. 29 A fragment of bone avulsed with the ulnar collateral ligament.

5 / Tendon injuries

Cut flexor tendons

Division of a flexor tendon in the hand is a serious injury that is often associated with some permanent disability.

Clinical signs Tendons are usually divided by cuts from sharp objects and common mechanisms include grasping a knife blade, falling on broken glass or opening a can. It is a good rule when dealing with cuts on the hand to suspect that underlying structures have been divided until proved otherwise by surgical exploration.

Diagnosis Diagnosis is not usually difficult. When the outstretched hand is relaxed with the wrist extended the fingers normally make a 'cascade' with the degree of flexion increasing from index to little finger (Fig. 30). This posture is determined by the resting tone in the muscles and is altered if the deep flexor tendon or both flexor tendons are divided (Fig. 31) but not if only the superficialis tendon is cut.

The actions of both tendons should be tested and sensation and circulation in the finger checked because damage to the digital nerves and arteries is commonly associated.

Management Primary repair of flexor tendons should be done only by an expert. Between the distal palmar skin crease and the middle of the finger the tendons lie in the fibrous flexor sheath and cut tendons in this area are particularly difficult to deal with as dense adhesions will form after repair unless special techniques are used. Delayed tendon grafting is sometimes used to avoid this problem but primary repair by an expert is preferred.

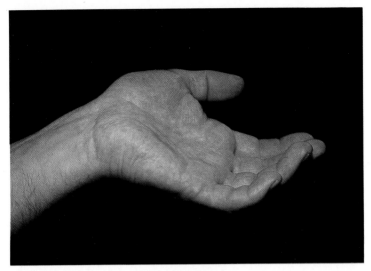
Fig. 30 Normal posture in the relaxed uninjured hand.

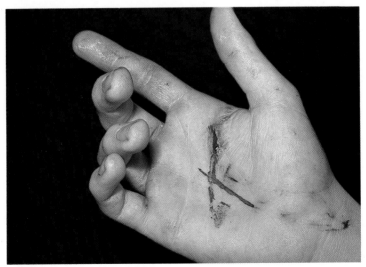
Fig. 31 The superficial and deep flexor tendons of the index finger have been cut in the palm.

Avulsion of flexor tendon

Mechanism   The metacarpophalangeal joint of the ring finger, which is almost invariably affected, has limited extension when the other fingers are flexed into the palm. The injury most often occurs when a rugby player grasps the shirt of another player and the ring finger is forcibly extended while the other fingers remain in the gripping position. The deep flexor tendon of the ring finger is avulsed from the terminal phalanx, preventing active flexion of the distal interphalangeal joint (Fig. 32), and may retract into the palm.

Management   Early surgical repair usually produces good results.

Extensor tendon injuries

The long extensor tendons on the wrist and back of the hand are usually damaged by sharp cutting injuries.

Clinical features   The patient is unable to extend the affected fingers at the metacarpophalangeal joints (Fig. 33). The interphalangeal joints can still be straightened by the intrinsic muscles acting on the intact extensor expansion of the fingers.

Management   Primary repair has a much better prognosis than in flexor tendon injuries but careful supervision is still necessary to obtain a good result. Tendon grafting or tendon transfer may be necessary in the late case.

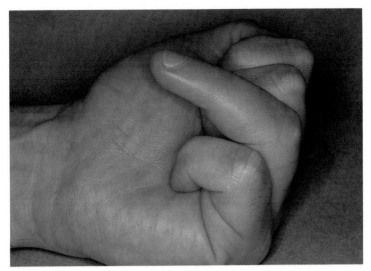

Fig. 32 Avulsion of the deep flexor tendon of the ring finger. Patient attempting to make a fist.

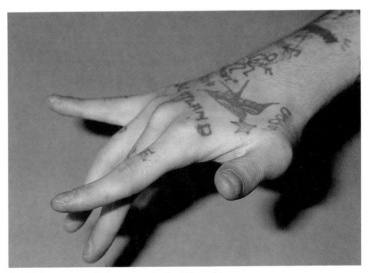

Fig. 33 Cut extensor digitorum communis at the wrist.

Mallet finger

A rupture of the extensor mechanism at its insertion into the terminal phalanx, often the result of a trivial flexion injury.

Clinical features   The distal phalanx cannot be extended actively and lies in about 20–60° of flexion (Fig. 34).

Management   The injured joint is kept extended in a plastic splint for about 6 weeks.

Boutonnière deformity

The result of rupture or division of the central slip of the extensor expansion on the dorsum of the proximal interphalangeal joint (PIPJ). The lateral bands of the expansion slip laterally and anteriorly, eventually coming to act as flexors of the PIPJ and causing hyperextension of the distal interphalangeal joint (DIPJ) (Fig. 35).

Management   Early splintage or surgical repair is necessary to prevent a fixed deformity.

Rupture of extensor pollicis longus tendon

Spontaneous rupture may occur after a Colles' fracture or when the wrist is affected by rheumatoid arthritis.

Clinical features   The patient may feel something snap and is then unable to extend the thumb (Fig. 36).

Management   Transfer of the extensor indicis proprius tendon to the distal part of the ruptured tendon.

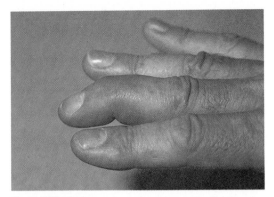

Fig. 34 Mallet finger.

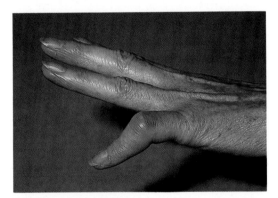

Fig. 35 Boutonnière deformity.

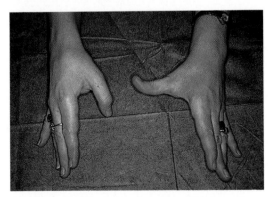

Fig. 36 Rupture of the tendon of extensor pollicis longus in the right hand.

6 / **Nerve injuries**

The hand is supplied by the median and ulnar nerves, which contain both motor and sensory fibres, and the radial nerve which supplies sensation to the radial border of the back of the hand.

Nerves are commonly divided when the hand is cut and injury to an underlying nerve must always be suspected. Nerve repair should be carried out by an expert. Full recovery is not always achieved after repair of mixed nerves in adults but useful functional recovery is gained in many cases.

Median nerve

Function   The median nerve in the hand supplies the abductor pollicis brevis, the opponens pollicis, the radial two lumbricals and may give a motor supply to the flexor pollicis brevis muscle. It gives sensation to the skin over the thenar eminence, the palmar aspect of the thumb and the radial two and one half fingers. Variations in the motor and sensory supply are not uncommon and there is also overlap with adjacent sensory areas.

Clinical signs   When the median nerve is cut the patient is unable to abduct the thumb (Fig. 37). Wasting of the median innervated muscles will follow (Fig. 38).

Loss of function of the median nerve is very serious because the thumb cannot be positioned against the tips of the fingers and sensation is lost in the 'picking-up' area of the hand.

See also carpal tunnel syndrome (p. 95).

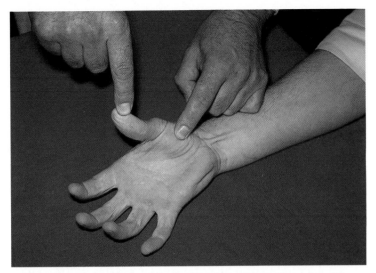

Fig. 37 Testing normal abduction of the thumb against resistance. Contraction of the muscles is visible and palpable.

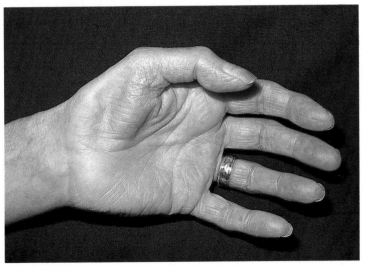

Fig. 38 Visible wasting of the abductor pollicis brevis muscle.

Ulnar nerve

Function The ulnar nerve supplies those intrinsic muscles of the hand that are not supplied by the median nerve: the adductor pollicis, the hypothenar muscles, the interossei and the ulnar two lumbricals. Flexor pollicis brevis often has a supply from both nerves and anatomical variations are not uncommon.

It supplies sensation to the palmar aspect of the little finger and the ulnar side of the ring finger and the back of the hand except for the area supplied by the radial nerve.

Clinical signs When the ulnar nerve is cut at the wrist there is wasting of the ulnar-innervated intrinsic muscles, most obviously the first dorsal interosseous and the little and ring finger adopt a position of flexion — the 'ulnar claw hand' (Fig. 39).

When the patient attempts to grip a flat object between the thumb and the hand, the flexor pollicis longus (innervated by the median nerve) comes into action to overcome the effects of the paralysis of adductor pollicis. The result is flexion of the interphalangeal joint of the thumb — Froment's sign (Fig. 40).

The patient is unable to grip a piece of paper between two fingers because the interossei are paralysed (Fig. 41). The hand must be kept flat when doing this test to avoid trick movements using the extrinsic muscles.

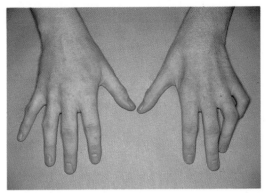

Fig. 39 Wasting of the first dorsal interosseous muscle and slight clawing of the ulnar two fingers in the left hand.

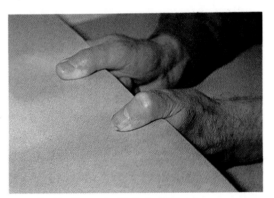

Fig. 40 Positive Froment's sign in the left hand.

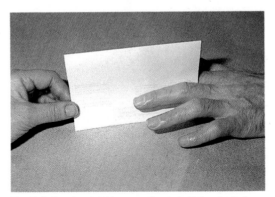

Fig. 41 Patient (on right) is attempting to hold the sheet of paper against a gentle pull from the examiner.

7 / Fingertip injuries

An apparently minor injury of the fingertip can be followed by marked disability unless treatment is carefully supervised.

The aim of treatment is to achieve early sound healing so that the patient may use the finger in normal activities.

Subungual haematoma

Description A collection of blood under the finger nail (Fig. 42), usually the result of a crushing injury, for example catching the finger in the door of a car.

Management There may be an associated fracture of the terminal phalanx but this can usually be ignored as it is well splinted by the nail.

In the acute phase the blood can be drained by drilling a couple of holes in the nail and this will greatly relieve discomfort.

Nail dislocation

Description This injury occurs in children when the epiphyseal plate at the base of the terminal phalanx is still open. A crushing injury produces a fracture dislocation through the plate, allowing the nail to displace (Figs 43 and 44).

Management The fracture is an open one and should be treated with great care to avoid infection. The nail should not be removed but returned to its bed so that it may stabilize the fracture and prevent adhesions forming between the layers of the nail fold. The distal joint is splinted for 2 weeks.

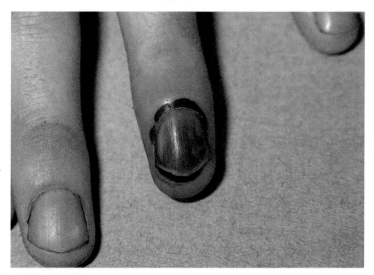

Fig. 42 Subungual haematoma.

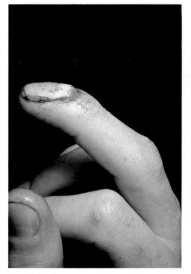

Fig. 43 Displacement of the nail from the nail fold.

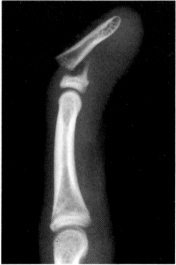

Fig. 44 The associated fracture of the terminal phalanx.

Partial amputations

Partial amputations are common industrial injuries (Fig. 45).

Management   The aim of treatment is to restore a pain–free fingertip with good sensation and stable skin cover.

Often the wound can be closed primarily if the terminal phalanx is trimmed. Alternatively the skin can be replaced using small local flaps. Small areas of skin loss without exposure of the bone can be allowed to heal secondarily, as can most fingertip injuries in children.

Complications   If most of the terminal phalanx has been lost there is no support for the nail and it may grow in a curled and unsightly way (Fig. 46). Ablation of the nail may be necessary.

Small remnants of the germinal matrix will continue to produce nail tissue which may form a mass of keratin (Fig. 47) or a spike of nail. The nail-forming tissue should be removed.

See also digital amputations (pp. 39–42).

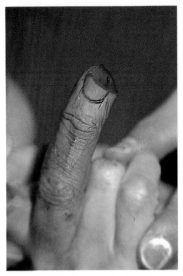

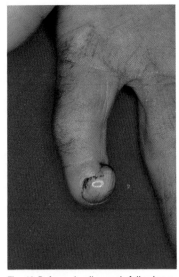

Fig. 45 A slicing injury of the fingertip.

Fig. 46 Deformed nail growth following a partial amputation of the fingertip.

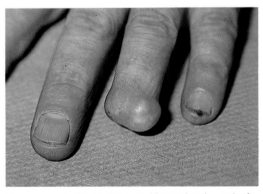

Fig. 47 A keratin–filled lesion caused by continued growth of nail remnants.

8 / Special types of injury

Major crush injuries

Major crush injuries (Fig. 48) are often due to
industrial accidents involving machinery such as
presses.

Management   Initial treatment consists of removing all dead tissue
and tissue of doubtful viability. Exposed tissues must
be covered with skin and this may require technically
difficult methods such as free flaps with microvascular
anastomoses.

Reconstructive procedures must be planned
individually for each patient, the aim being to provide
a hand with sensation and the ability to grip.

Wringer injuries

Wringer or roller injuries cause crushing of all
structures in the hand and the skin may be stripped
off underlying structures.

Management   Distally based flaps (Fig. 49) are seldom viable and
should not be stitched back. Lost skin should be
replaced using appropriate grafts or flaps.

Guillotine injuries

Clean cut amputations (Fig. 50) and those with
minimal crushing are suitable for replantation using
microsurgical techniques.

Management   The amputated part should be sealed in a sterile
plastic bag, placed on ordinary ice and sent with the
patient without delay to a centre with microsurgical
facilities.

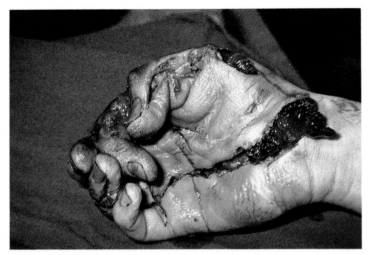
Fig. 48 Crushing injury caused by a book-binding press.

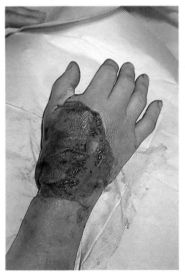
Fig. 49 Roller injury. Note that the skin flap is clearly dead.

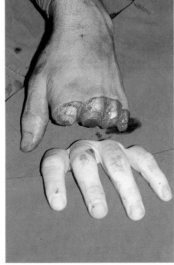
Fig. 50 Industrial guillotine injury.

Injection injuries

Injuries caused by high pressure injection guns may appear trivial (Fig. 51) but foreign material such as grease or paint is forced into the tissues of the hand and extensive necrosis will occur unless the material is removed promptly.

Management Early and wide exploration to remove all material.

Burns

Burns vary from the superficial to the extensive, deep burn (Fig. 52). A special category is the electrical burn which is nearly always much deeper than it appears.

Management The cornerstones of treatment are control of oedema, maintainence of movement and relief of pain. Excision of dead skin and replacement by skin grafting is necessary in deep burns.
   Further surgery may be needed to restore movement by tendon grafting or release of contractures. Expert rehabilitation is essential.

Frostbite

Cold injury can cause necrosis of the fingertips (Fig. 53) or more extensive damage.

Management In the acute phase the whole patient should be warmed and the damaged parts thawed in a waterbath. The role of vasodilator and anticoagulating drugs is unclear. Amputation should be delayed until there is clear demarcation between living and dead tissue.

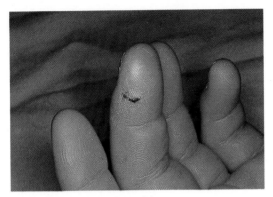

Fig. 51 High pressure greasegun injury.

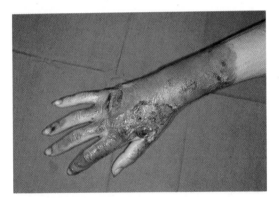

Fig. 52 A deep burn of the hand.

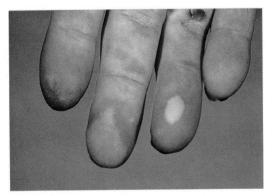

Fig. 53 Frostbite affecting the fingertips.

9 / Self–inflicted injuries

Slashed wrist

'Wrist–slashing' is common. It may be an attention–seeking gesture or a serious attempt at suicide. Considerable damage may be caused to deeper stuctures even when this was not intended.

Clinical features

Typically there are several cuts which vary in depth (Fig. 54). Assessment of the extent of damage may be difficult as the patient is often uncooperative.

Management

All patients should be assessed by a psychiatrist. If there is any doubt about the extent of injury the wrist should be explored when the patient's condition allows and divided structures repaired. Rehabilitation may be difficult and the wrist–slashing may be repeated.

Dermatitis artefacta

The possibility of self–inflicted injury should be considered when a patient has odd skin lesions that show no specific abnormality on biopsy and which fail to heal despite various treatments.

Clinical features

Dermatitis artefacta may take many forms such as repeated scratching with some object or cigarette burns (Fig. 55).

Management

Lesions often heal if the area is kept occluded but the patient will often remove dressings or casts for seemingly plausible reasons. Even when it is obvious that the lesion is self–inflicted it may be blandly denied, but psychiatric assessment may elicit a reason for this type of behaviour.

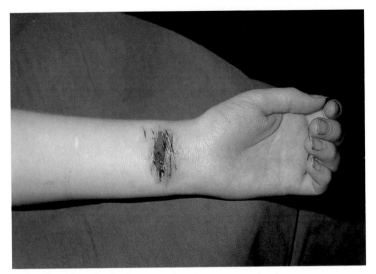

Fig. 54 A typical slashed wrist.

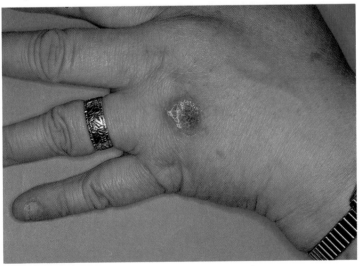

Fig. 55 Dermatitis artefacta. The lesion was due to a cigarette burn.

10 / **Digital amputations**

Digital amputations may be the result of severe injury or may be required for infection, malignant disease or severe deformity, for example due to Dupuytren's disease (p. 75).

Index finger

If the amputation causes significant shortening, the stump of the index finger is of little use and tends to be bypassed when making a pinch grip (Fig. 56).

Management   Amputation through the metacarpophalangeal joint leaves an unsightly projection caused by the metacarpal head; an oblique amputation through the metacarpal shaft gives a better cosmetic result (Fig. 57).

Middle and ring fingers

The ideal level of proximal amputation is debatable. Small objects slip from the hand if the finger is removed at the metacarpophalangeal joint.

Management   This problem can be helped by leaving a small stump of the finger (Fig. 58). The gap between the fingers can be lessened by removing the finger and its metacarpal bone (ray amputation).

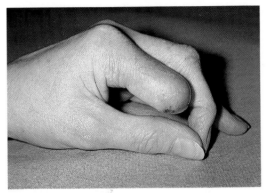

Fig. 56 A short stump of the index finger is not used when gripping small objects.

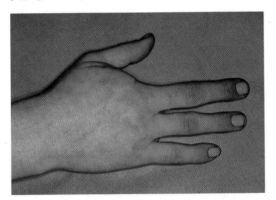

Fig. 57 The appearance of the hand after amputation of the index finger through the metacarpal bone.

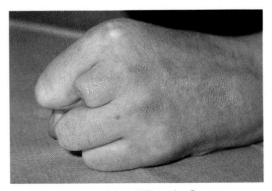

Fig. 58 A small stump of the middle or ring finger may prevent small objects slipping from the palm.

Little finger

The little and ring fingers are important for stabilizing objects gripped strongly in the hand. A weak power grip results when the little finger or both of these fingers have been lost (Fig. 59) or cannot be flexed into the palm because of stiffness. Even a small stump of the little finger helps in power grip, provided it is mobile, and should be retained if possible.

Thumb

The ability to oppose the thumb to the fingers is of supreme importance in the function of the hand. Complete loss of the thumb is a major injury as the hand can function only as a paddle or hook.

Every effort should be made to preserve functional length of the thumb in partial amputations (Fig. 60), although tightly stretched, unstable skin over the stump should be avoided.

Management   Microsurgical replantation of a traumatically amputated thumb should be performed if circumstances are favourable. If this is not possible secondary procedures to reconstruct a new thumb will be necessary. Several types of procedures have been devised including the transfer of a toe to the hand, construction of a thumb from the index finger (pollicization) and lengthening the thumb metacarpal bone to provide an opposition post.

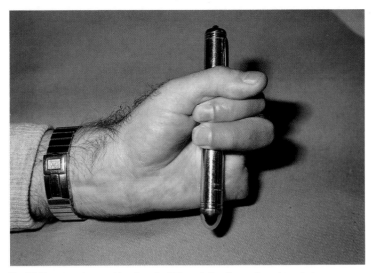

Fig. 59 The grasp is unstable when the little and ring fingers have been lost.

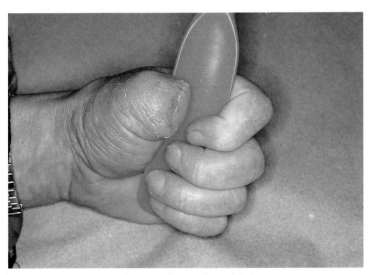

Fig. 60 Even a short length of thumb is functionally useful.

11 / Congenital anomalies

Congenital anomalies may affect only the hand or be part of a malformation syndrome or skeletal dysplasia.

Aetiology A congenital anomaly may be inherited or sporadic. The latter may be due to damage during development (e.g. thalidomide deformities). Often no cause is found.

Classification
- Failure of formation
- Failure of separation
- Duplication
- Overgrowth
- Undergrowth
- Constriction bands
- Miscellaneous
- Associated with generalized skeletal abnormalities

Management Treatment may not be necessary but if so should be directed to improving function rather than cosmesis. Major reconstructive procedures should be completed before school age if possible.

Failure of formation

Transverse Distal transverse defects are usually sporadic (non–hereditary). The upper third of the forearm is a common site (Fig. 61) and early prosthetic fitting is helpful.

Children with distal transverse defects in the hand (Fig. 62) often have excellent function if the other hand is normal.

Longitudinal A typical example would be failure of formation of the radius producing a radial club hand (Fig. 63). Treatment aims to provide a useful hand in a functional position, by centralizing the hand on the radius and constructing a thumb from the index finger (pollicization). The elbow must be mobile or the child will not be able to reach the mouth.

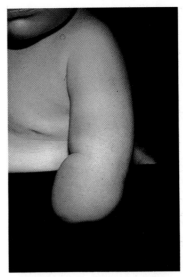

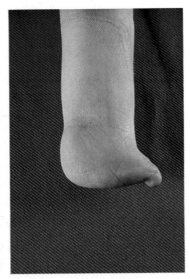

Fig. 61 Transverse deficit of the forearm.

Fig. 62 A distal transverse deficit.

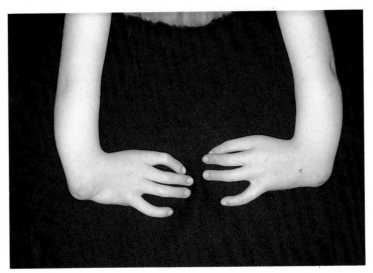

Fig. 63 Radial club hands.

Failure of separation

Examples **Syndactyly** (incomplete separation of the digits): may be an isolated anomaly or part of a generalized malformation syndrome. Pattern of inheritance is variable.

Simple syndactyly: the fingers are joined, either partially or completely, by skin alone (Fig. 64). They can be separated by relatively simple plastic surgical procedures with expectation of a good cosmetic and functional result.

Complex syndactyly: both skin and bone are joined. Surgical treatment is difficult but worthwhile.

Acrosyndactyly: the fingers are joined distally, leaving a space between the fingers more proximally. In Apert's syndrome complex bilateral syndactyly (Fig. 65) is associated with characteristic craniofacial abnormalities.

Duplication

Example **Polydactyly**: the possession of extra digits (Fig. 66), is fairly common. It may be an isolated hand abnormality or occur as part of a congenital malformation syndrome with variable inheritance.

Management An obviously abnormal and functionless digit should be removed.

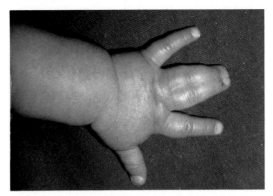

Fig. 64 Simple syndactyly.

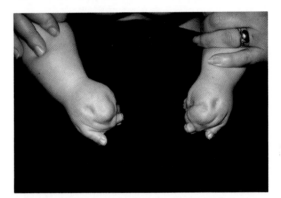

Fig. 65 Complex syndactyly in Apert's syndrome.

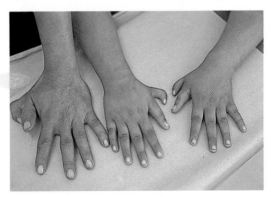

Fig. 66 Bilateral pre-axial polydactyly. The other hand belongs to the patient's father.

Overgrowth

Example   ***Macrodactyly***: localized gigantism of a digit.

Clinical features   Macrodactyly is usually unilateral, affecting one or more digits (Fig. 67) and apparent within the first 2 years of life. All tissues in the fingers are involved.

Management   Treatment is difficult. Local resection of the involved tissue is not always successful and amputation may be necessary if the appearance of the finger is bizarre and it has no function.

Undergrowth

Example   ***Metacarpal shortening***: most often affects the little and ring finger rays (Fig. 68). It is usually transmitted as an autosomal dominant trait.

Management   There is no significant functional deficit and treatment is not required.

Constriction bands

Definition   Annular grooves at right angles to the long axis of the limb which may be completely circumferential. Their occurrence is sporadic and their cause is not established.

Clinical features   Range from intra-uterine amputation to a small groove on a finger (Fig. 69). Acrosyndactyly (p. 45) is common.

Management   Tight constriction bands should be resected and acrosyndactyly should be separated.

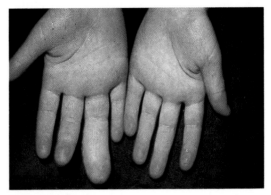

Fig. 67 Macrodactyly.

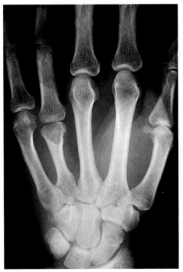

Fig. 68 A short metacarpal bone.

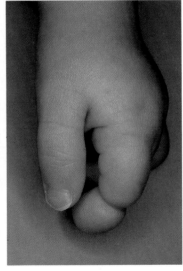

Fig. 69 Constriction band.

Generalized skeletal disorders

In these disorders the hand abnormality is a manifestation of a condition that also affects other parts of the skeleton. There is a large number of such conditions although they are relatively uncommon. A few of the more common will be described.

Diaphyseal aclasis (multiple exostoses)

Clinical features Palpable and often visible osteocartilaginous outgrowths most common around knees, ankles and shoulders. Lumps in the hand may produce deformities and interfere with function if they are near joints (Figs 70 and 71). Inherited as autosomal dominant.

Management Removal of unsightly exostoses or those affecting function.

Multiple enchondromatosis (Ollier's disease)

Clinical features The condition is characterized by the persistence of unmineralized cartilage within long bones usually with asymmetrical involvement. Large and unsightly cartilaginous tumours may occur in the hands (Figs 72 and 73). Malignant change can occur. Sporadic in occurrence with no genetic basis.

Management Amputation of severely involved and functionally useless parts.

See also enchondroma (p. 71).

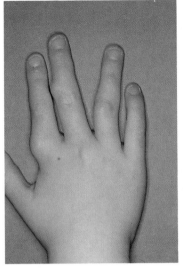

Fig. 70 Diaphyseal aclasis.

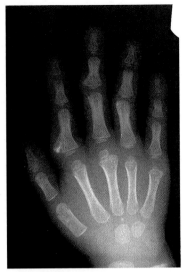

Fig. 71 Diaphyseal aclasis.

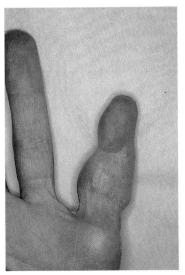

Fig. 72 Ollier's disease.

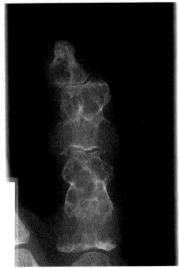

Fig. 73 Ollier's disease.

Generalized skeletal disorders (contd)

Marfan's syndrome

Clinical features
A generalized connective tissue disorder inherited as an autosomal dominant trait. Characterized by tall, slender build, aortic dilatation and incompetence and dislocation of the lenses of the eyes. The hands are typically long and thin (Figs 74 and 75), hence the alternative name of *arachnodactyly* for the condition.

Management
Treatment is not required as the hands are functionally normal.

Achondroplasia

Clinical features
A relatively common condition of autosomal dominant inheritance, in which the limbs are short but growth of the trunk and head is almost normal. The hands ('trident hands') are short and broad (Fig. 76).

Management
Treatment is not required as the hands are functionally normal.

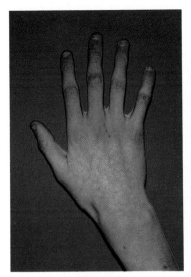

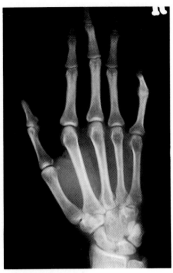

Fig. 74 Marfan's syndrome.

Fig. 75 Marfan's syndrome.

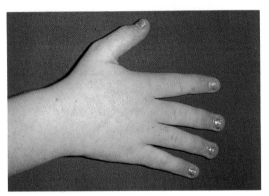

Fig. 76 Achondroplasia.

Miscellaneous abnormalities

Many congenital hand disorders are not readily classified in the groups already described. Some examples will be given.

Camptodactyly

Clinical features
Presents as a flexion contracture of the proximal interphalangeal joints, most often affecting the little fingers (Fig. 77). It is usually of autosomal dominant inheritance but may be sporadic.

Management
Treatment is usually not required. It is difficult to improve the fingers by either splintage or surgery.

Clinodactyly

Clinical features
A lateral curvature of the little finger caused by asymmetrical growth of the intermediate phalanx (Fig. 78). It is usually of autosomal dominant inheritance.

Management
Treatment is rarely required, although corrective osteotomy may be required in severe cases.

Triphalangeal thumb

Clinical features
The thumb has an extra phalanx and in some cases the digit may have the appearance and movements of a finger — the 'five-fingered hand' (Fig. 79). This may be of autosomal dominant inheritance.

Management
Pollicization of the radial digit.

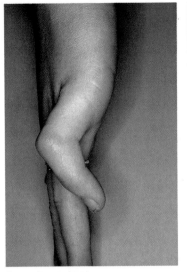

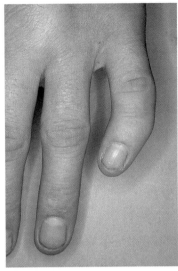

Fig. **77** Camptodactyly.

Fig. **78** Clinodactyly.

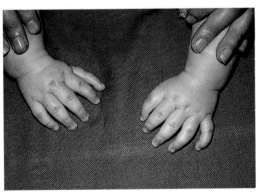

Fig. **79** Five-fingered hands.

12 / **Infections**

The classic bacterial hand infections described in many textbooks are now seldom seen, perhaps because of early treatment with antibiotics; nevertheless, infections can still severely damage the hand unless treated early and well. The essentials of treatment are splintage and elevation of the hand, adequate surgical drainage of localized pus and appropriate antibiotic therapy. Staphylococci are the organisms most commonly isolated.

Pulp space

Pulp space infections (Fig. 80) often follow minor injuries.

Clinical features   The fingertip is swollen and painful and the patient suffers from a throbbing pain that prevents sleep.

Management   If the infection does not settle rapidly with antibiotic therapy, surgical drainage should be performed before there is damage to skin or bone.

Paronychia

Infection of the nail fold (Fig. 81) is one of the more common hand infections.

Clinical features   Redness, swelling and pain localized to the base of the nail. The infection may track completely round the nail.

Management   Localized pus should be released from under the nail by removal of a corner of the nail at the germinal fold.

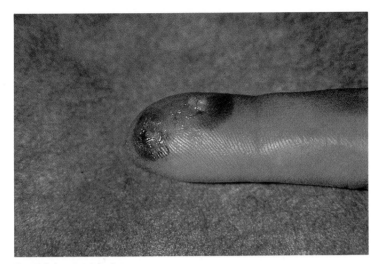

Fig. 80 Pulp space infection.

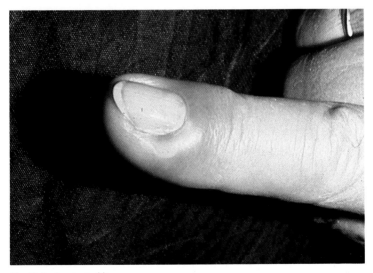

Fig. 81 Acute paronychia

Web space

Infection in the loose tissue between the digits may
follow minor skin trauma.

Clinical
features

Infection is usually well–localized between the digits.
There is marked swelling, pain and pointing of pus
may be seen (Fig. 82).

Management

Pus should be adequately drained without delay and
an appropriate antibiotic started.

Tendon sheath

Infection of the tendon sheath usually follows a
penetrating injury, although this may be so minor that
it is forgotten. Bites can cause particularly severe
infections.

Clinical
features

The finger is slightly swollen and reddened (Fig. 83).
There is tenderness over the line of the fibrous flexor
sheath. Active movement of the finger is prevented by
pain which is increased by attempted passive
movement.

Management

Early antibiotic treatment may mask the severity of
the infection. The tendon sheath should be drained
and irrigated if the ability to move the finger does not
return rapidly. Delay in surgical treatment may result
in necrosis of the tendon and a stiff, useless finger.

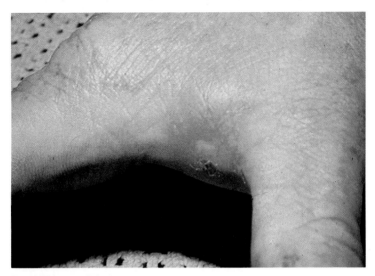

Fig. 82 Web space infection.

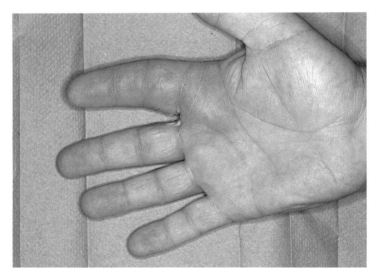

Fig. 83 Tendon sheath infection.

Septic arthritis

Septic arthritis is usually caused by a fist fight. The knuckles strike the teeth of an opponent and organisms from the mouth enter the metacarpophalangeal joint. As the hand relaxes the extensor tendon expansion seals the joint, preventing drainage of infected material.

Clinical features Treatment is usually sought a few days after the injury. There is severe pain and inability to move the finger. On examination there is a puncture wound or cut over the joint, usually surrounded by cellulitis (Fig. 84).

Management Early exploration and drainage of the joint is required before the infection destroys the articular surface (Fig. 85). The bacteria involved are commonly anaerobic and appropriate antibiotics should be given.

Pyogenic granuloma

Although this lesion is often stated to be a proliferative response to a trivial infection, it may be a variety of capillary haemangioma (p. 69).

Clinical features A painful red tumour that bleeds easily, usually on the palmar aspect of the hand (Fig. 86).

Management Treatment is by surgical excision, taking care to remove all the involved tissue.

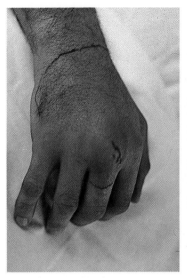

Fig. 84 Septic arthritis of a metacarpophalangeal joint.

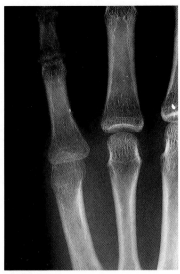

Fig. 85 Spontaneous ankylosis after septic arthritis.

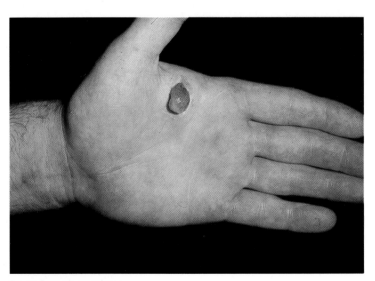

Fig. 86 Pyogenic granuloma.

Warts

The hand is a frequent site for the common wart (*verruca vulgaris*) (Fig. 87). They may be isolated or multiple and are caused by a papova DNA virus.

Management   Many disappear spontaneously, otherwise they can be removed by curettage or cryotherapy using liquid nitrogen.

Orf

A viral disease of sheep and goats.

Clinical features   The infection occurs in people handling the carcasses of infected animals. Lesions occur most often on the hand or forearm. Initially papular, they become vesicular and later pustular (Fig. 88). They are not accompanied by a systemic illness.

Management   Treatment is not usually necessary as this is a self–limiting condition resolving in a few weeks.

Herpetic whitlow

Infection with type I herpes simplex virus. Secretions from infected people enter the skin through abrasions. Common in nurses, dentists and medical staff.

Clinical features   Painful vesicular lesions on a digit (Fig. 89). Painful recurrence is common.

Management   Antiviral agents may shorten the attack but do not necessarily prevent recurrence.

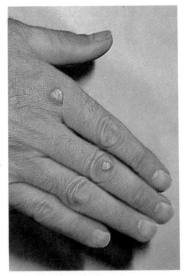

Fig. 87 Common warts.

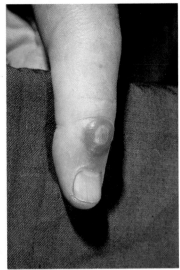

Fig. 88 Orf.

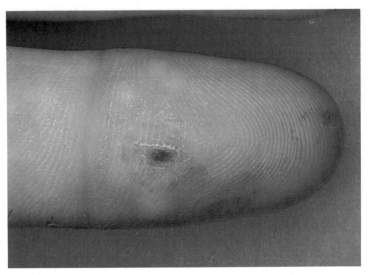

Fig. 89 Herpetic whitlow.

Erysipeloid

Infection by *Erysipelothrix insidiosa* occurring in those who handle raw meat and fish. The organism may gain entrance through a scratch.

Clinical features Slowly spreading cellulitis affecting usually one finger (Fig. 90), without significant pain or constitutional features.

Management Erysipeloid tends to resolve slowly without treatment. Penicillin or tetracycline are effective.

Scabies

Infection by *Sarcoptes scabiei hominis*, a burrowing mite, which is spread by close contact.

Clinical features The hand and wrist are common sites. The lesions are itchy when warm, e.g. in bed. Secondary changes due to scratching are common (Fig. 91). The burrow can be seen under magnification.

Management Patients and their close contacts should be treated with gamma benzene hexachloride cream or benzyl benzoate which should be applied to the whole body below the neck.

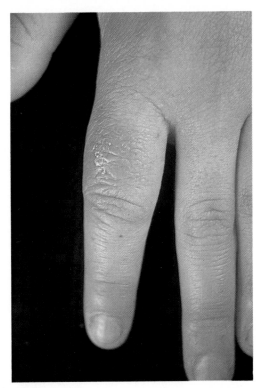

Fig. 90 Erysipeloid.

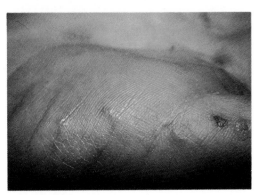

Fig. 91 Scabies.

13 / **Benign tumours**

Included under this heading are some lesions that are not true neoplasms but which present as swellings in the hand.

Ganglion

Pathology

A cystic lesion with a fibrous capsule containing viscous material similar to synovial fluid. The cause is unknown.

Clinical features

Ganglions are very common, with peak incidence in young adults. The most common site is the dorsum of the wrist (Fig. 92) but they also occur on the flexor aspect of the wrist, in association with the fibrous flexor sheaths or as cysts within carpal bones.

Management

Most wrist ganglions resolve spontaneously. Treatment is indicated if the lesion is unsightly or causes local discomfort. Recurrence is common after surgical excision. Aspiration and multiple puncture, repeated if necessary, is as effective.

Epidermoid inclusion cyst

Pathogenesis

A trivial injury resulting in subcutaneous implantation of a piece of keratinized skin which continues to grow and forms a cyst lined with squamous epithelium and which contains cholesterol–rich fluid.

Clinical features

Presents as a firm, painless swelling on the volar aspect of the hand (Fig. 93).

Management

Excision.

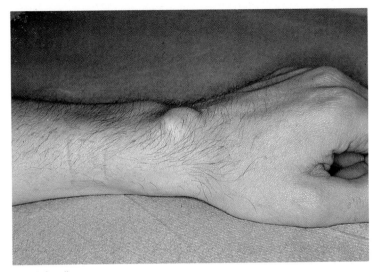

Fig. 92 Ganglion.

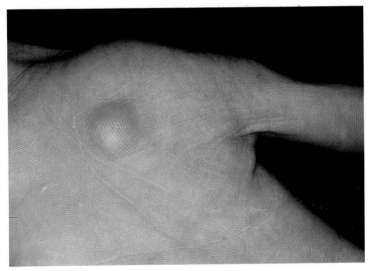

Fig. 93 Epidermoid cyst in palm.

Lipoma

Pathology   Proliferation of fat cells.

Clinical   A rather uncommon tumour in the hand, although
features   common elsewhere in the upper limb.
 Presents as a painless, soft swelling, usually in the
 palm (Fig. 94). The extent of the lesion may be
 masked if it lies deep to the unyielding palmar fascia.

Management   Surgical removal.

Pigmented villonodular synovitis (PVNS)

Synonyms   Giant cell tumour of tendon sheath; fibrous xanthoma
 of synovium.

Pathology   PVNS may be a true tumour but probably represents
 a reaction to trauma or infection.
 The lesion is yellowy-grey due to lipid and
 haemosiderin. It may be locally infiltrative.
 Histologically it contains histiocytes and multinucleate
 macrophages.

Clinical   A relatively common tumour in middle age.
features   Usually presents as a painless, firm swelling on the
 flexor aspect of a digit (Fig. 95), although it may
 arise from the dorsal aspect of the terminal
 interphalangeal joint.

Management   Excision. Recurrence may follow if this is incomplete.

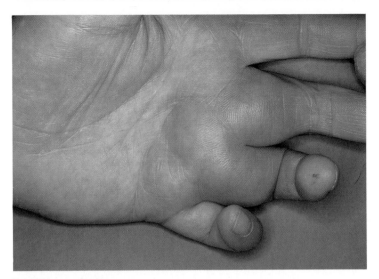

Fig. 94 Lipoma of palm.

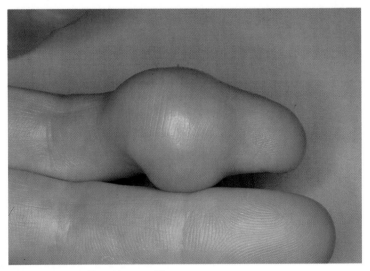

Fig. 95 Pigmented villonodular synovitis.

Glomus tumour

Pathology   A well–defined, encapsulated lesion arising from the glomus body, a collection of anastomosing blood vessels surrounded by nerves and epithelioid cells. Histologically the tumour is highly vascular and contains many nerve endings.

Clinical features   An uncommon tumour which presents as an exquisitely tender area at the tip of the finger which is extremely sensitive to heat and cold.

50% of glomus tumours are subungual. There may be no visible abnormality but sometimes a bluish discoloration can be seen under the nail or the lunula may be distorted (Fig. 96). Radiographs sometimes show scalloping of the terminal phalanx (Fig. 97) — a common finding when there is any tumour at the tip of the finger.

Management   Excision. Recurrence may occur if this is incomplete.

Haemangioma/vascular malformation

Pathology   A *haemangioma* is a local tumour of blood vessels that commonly develops in the first year of life. *Vascular malformations* vary from capillary blemishes (Fig. 98) to large lesions that extend through several tissue planes and may be associated with arteriovenous fistulae and localized overgrowth.

Management   True haemangiomas often regress spontaneously. Vascular malformations may be impossible to remove surgically because of their complexity.

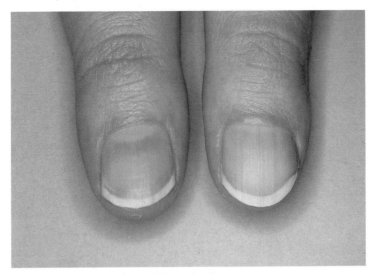

Fig. 96 A glomus tumour under the left thumb nail.

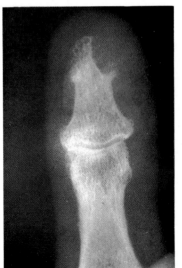

Fig. 97 Scalloping of a terminal phalanx.

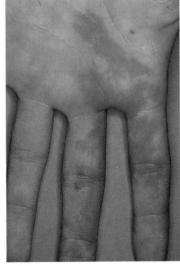

Fig. 98 A capillary vascular malformation.

Enchondroma

Pathology An enchondroma is the most common bone tumour in the hand. It is thought to arise from cartilage cells left in long bones during development.

Usually centrally placed in metacarpal bones or phalanges and most often solitary, but multiple in Ollier's disease (p. 49). The tumour does not increase in size when skeletal growth has ceased. Malignant change is very rare in solitary enchondromata.

Clinical features Usually found in adolescents and young adults, enchondromata may present as hard, painless swellings (Fig. 99) but often only come to light because of a pathological fracture (Fig. 100).

Radiographs show a circumscribed lytic lesion expanding the bone and often containing irregular flecks of calcification. Occasionally the lesion is not centrally placed — this type of tumour is called an *ecchondroma* (Fig. 101).

Management Treatment is not needed for asymptomatic lesions that are found by chance.

However, the lesion should be treated by thorough curettage if it is large and unsightly or the diagnosis is in doubt. Bone grafting is rarely required.

Fractures through enchondromata usually heal well and may be followed by disappearance of the tumour. A recurrent fracture is an indication for surgical treatment of the tumour.

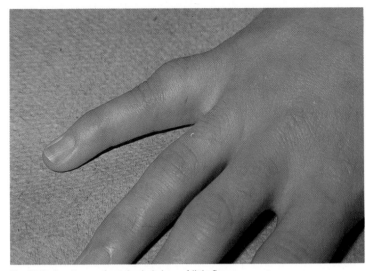

Fig. 99 Enchondroma of proximal phalanx of little finger.

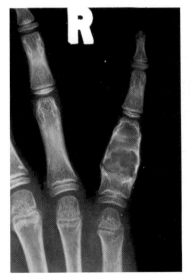

Fig. 100 A fracture through an enchondroma.

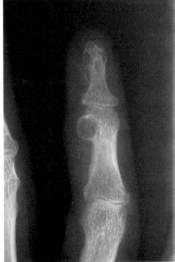

Fig. 101 An ecchondroma.

14 / Malignant tumours

Malignant tumours of the hand are quite rare.
Primary and secondary malignant bone tumours are
particularly uncommon, the most frequent lesions
being malignant tumours of the skin.

Squamous carcinoma

Squamous carcinomas are the most common
malignant tumour of the hand. Aetiological factors
include excessive exposure to sunlight, X-rays and
agents such as coal tar and oils.

Clinical features Usually presents as an ulcerative or cauliflower–like
lesion on the back of the hand (Fig. 102) that may
arise in an area of pre–existing hyperkeratosis. Spread
to regional nodes occurs in about 15% of cases.

Management Wide excision and skin grafting, or radiotherapy.

Malignant melanoma

Clinical features This tumour is relatively uncommon in the hand, the
most common site being the thumb.
  The tumour may be pigmented or amelanotic. It is
often subungual or in the nail fold (Fig. 103). It may
mimic a chronically infected lesion and should be
suspected if such a lesion does not respond rapidly to
antibiotic treatment. Local and distant spread is
common and can occur early.

Management Biopsy to confirm the diagnosis, followed by local
amputation. Immuno-, radio- and chemotherapy may
be used in conjunction.

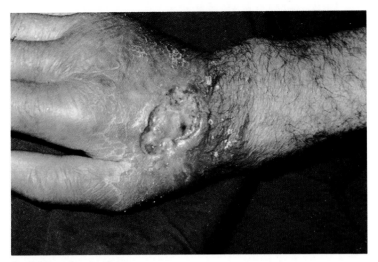

Fig. 102 Squamous carcinoma.

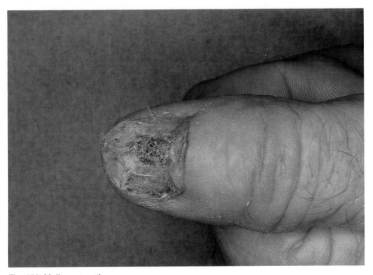

Fig. 103 Malignant melanoma.

15 / Dupuytren's disease

A disorder in which the palmar fascia becomes thickened and sometimes contracted.

Aetiology There is a strong hereditary element: the tendency to develop the disorder is transmitted as an autosomal dominant trait of variable penetrance. The disease is sometimes associated with others such as epilepsy, diabetes, alcoholism and cirrhosis of the liver. The significance of such associations is not clear.

It is not caused by injury or occupation, but injury may accelerate the onset of the condition in those predisposed to it.

Pathology Aggregates of contractile fibroblasts form in the palmar and digital fascia. Increased mitosis is seen in the active phase.

Incidence Dupuytren's disease is common in people of Northern European descent, but very rare in other races. A disease of middle and old age, present in up to 25% of men over the age of 65. Less common in women and only occasionally seen in young people.

Clinical features The earliest feature is often a thickening or nodule in the palmar fascia (Fig. 104), without contracture. Further involvement and contracture of the fascia prevents full extension of the finger (Fig. 105), although the ability to flex is maintained. The little and ring fingers are most often affected.

Knuckle pads (Garrod's pads) are sometimes found on the dorsum of the proximal interphalangeal joints (Fig. 106, p. 78). They are often uncomfortable when they first appear. Knuckle pads usually occur in young adults with a strong family history before there is any sign of the disease elsewhere.

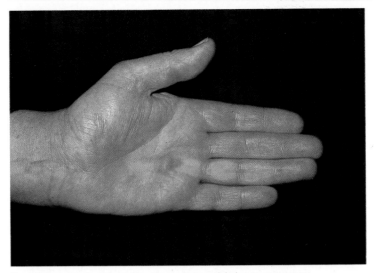

Fig. 104 Dupuytren's disease. There is a palmar nodule but no contracture.

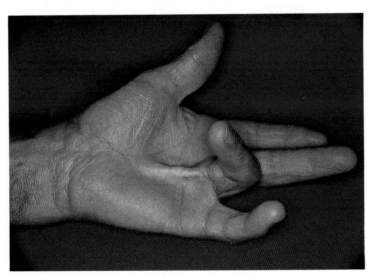

Fig. 105 A single band producing a contracture of the ring finger.

Management Treatment depends on the severity and progress of the disease.

Knuckle pads and palmar thickening without contractures do not need treatment.

Contractures may be static or increasing and their progress is unpredictable. A significant or rapidly increasing contracture are indications for treatment.

Exercise, splinting and massage have no effect on the rate of increase of the contracture.

Fasciectomy (excision of involved fascia) is the main form of treatment. Fasciotomy (simple division of fascial bands) may have a place in the treatment of single bands in elderly patients.

A contracture of the metacarpophalangeal joint can almost always be corrected completely by surgery. When the interphalangeal joints are involved (Fig. 107) secondary contractures in the capsular ligaments (p. 3) usually prevent full correction.

Recurrence or extension of the disease may occur after surgery (Fig. 108). Amputation of severely contracted fingers may be warranted when there is recurrent disease.

Carefully supervised physiotherapy is essential after operations for Dupuytren's disease.

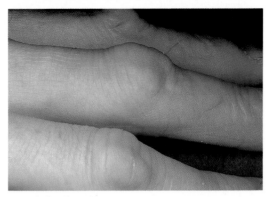

Fig. 106 Knuckle pads.

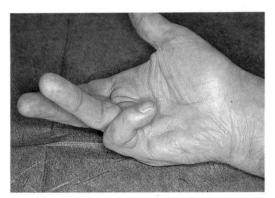

Fig. 107 Contractures at metacarpophalangeal and interphalangeal joints.

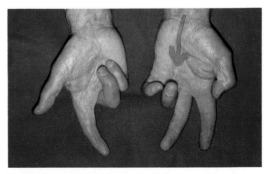

Fig. 108 Severe bilateral involvement after several operations including amputation.

16 / **Rheumatoid arthritis**

Definition   An inflammatory arthropathy of unknown aetiology which typically affects small joints in a symmetrical fashion at first, but larger joints may be affected by those with chronic disease.

Incidence   Common. More frequent in young and middle-aged women.

Pathology   Synovial proliferation produces swelling of the joints, stretching of ligaments and damage to tendons. Articular cartilage is covered with a pannus that destroys the joint surface.

Clinical features   Typical features are pain, swelling and stiffness. Thickened synovium may be palpated in flexor compartment of the fingers by the 'pinch test' (Figs 109 and 110).

Systemic symptoms such as malaise, weakness and loss of weight are often present.

Progression of the disease can lead to gross damage to joints and soft tissue in the hand, resulting in severe deformity and loss of function (Fig. 111).

Management   Initially by anti–inflammatory and analgesic drugs, rest and splintage.

Surgical treatment is aimed to restore function rather than improve the appearance of the hand, although that is often a secondary bonus. Very careful assessment of the patient's medical, physical and social problems is required before embarking on reconstructive surgical treatment.

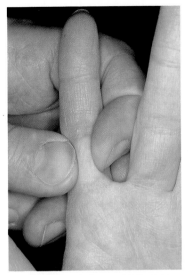

Fig. 109 Normal pinch test. A fold of skin can be pinched easily by the examiner.

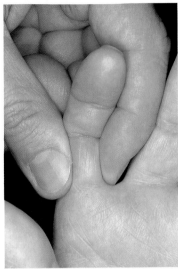

Fig. 110 When the test is positive a fold cannot be pinched.

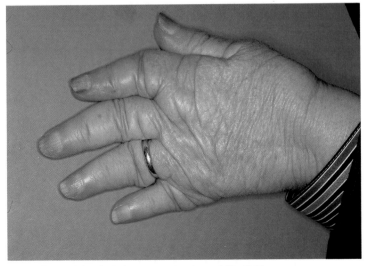

Fig. 111 Severe deformity in late progressive rheumatoid arthritis.

Some common problems in the hand caused by rheumatoid arthritis will be illustrated.

Dorsal synovitis

The wrist is commonly affected by the inflammatory processes of rheumatoid arthritis.

Description   Proliferative synovium arises from the synovial sheaths around tendons and the wrist joint itself.

Clinical features   The abnormal synovium on the dorsum of the wrist is usually visible and palpable. A constriction in the middle of the swelling caused by the extensor retinaculum results in an 'hour-glass' appearance (Fig. 112).

Management   Pain on extending the fingers and thumb in the presence of dorsal synovitis is an indication that rupture of the extensor tendons is impending. Surgical decompression or removal of the synovium may be necessary to prevent this.

Rupture of extensor tendons

Rupture more often occurs in the tendons on the ulnar side of the wrist (Fig. 113) and the extensor pollicis longus.

Mechanism   The tendons may be damaged by synovial proliferation or, in the case of the ulnar extensors, by attrition on the head of the ulnar which is commonly dislocated dorsally.

Management   Treatment is by excision of head of the ulna and reconstruction of extensor tendons.

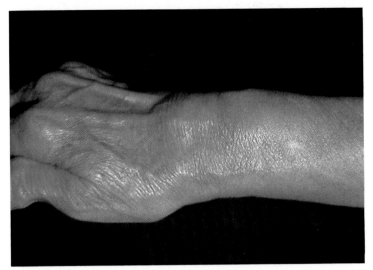

Fig. 112 Proliferative synovium under the extensor retinaculum.

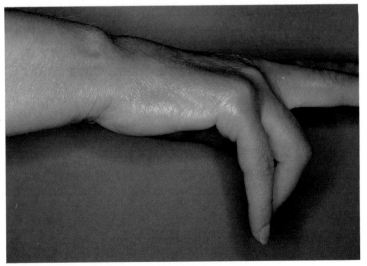

Fig. 113 Rupture of the extensor tendons to the ulnar fingers.

Ulnar drift

Ulnar deviation of the fingers is one of the characteristic deformities in the rheumatoid hand (Fig. 114).

Mechanism   Its pathogenesis is complex but it is partly attributable to synovitis in the metacarpophalangeal joints which stretches the collateral ligaments and causes displacement of the extensor tendons to the ulnar side of the metacarpal heads.

Management   Corrective surgery is directed to obtaining stability at the metacarpophalangeal joints, usually by the use of silicone rubber hinge implants, and realigning the pull of the tendons.

Thumb deformities

Many varieties of deformity of the thumb are caused by rheumatoid arthritis. A common type is the 'Z' deformity in which the thumb is flexed at the metacarpophalangeal joint and extended at the interphalangeal joint (Fig. 115). An adduction contracture of the first web space may also be present.

Mechanism   Synovitis in the metacarpophalangeal joint alters the action of the extensor tendons and intrinsic muscles acting on the thumb.

Management   Stabilization of the metacarpophalangeal joint will usually improve the function of the thumb.

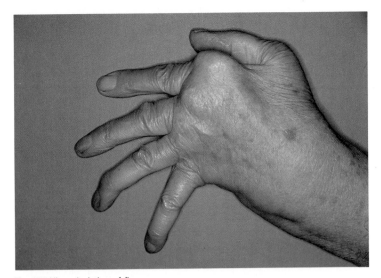

Fig. 114 Ulnar deviation of fingers.

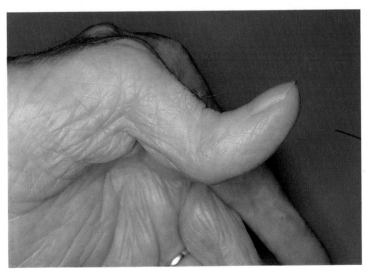

Fig. 115 'Z' deformity of thumb.

Swan neck deformity

The finger is held in hyperextension at the proximal interphalangeal joint and flexion at the distal interphalangeal joint (Fig. 116).

Mechanism Like most rheumatoid deformities it is the result of imbalance in the actions of muscles that follows the destruction of joints and stretching of ligaments and tendons by proliferative synovium.

The deformity may follow rupture or stretching of the extensor on the dorsum of the distal interphalangeal joint, which initially produces a mallet finger deformity (p. 23). Alternatively it may be secondary to stretching of the volar plate of the proximal interphalangeal joint. It is a fairly constant 'rule' in rheumatoid arthritis that joints adjacent to a deformed joint tend to develop the opposite deformity.

Boutonnière deformity

The finger is held in flexion at the proximal interphalangeal joint and hyperextension at the distal interphalangeal joint (Fig. 117).

Mechanism The pathogenesis of this deformity is described on page 23. In rheumatoid arthritis the central slip of the extensor tendon is damaged on the dorsum of the proximal interphalangeal joint by proliferative synovium arising from the joint.

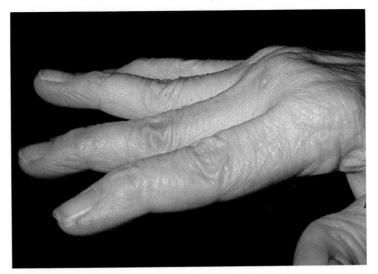

Fig. 116 Swan neck deformity.

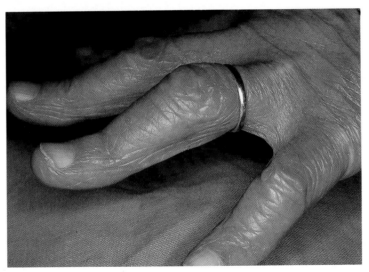

Fig. 117 Boutonnière deformity.

17 / **Osteoarthritis**

Although primary osteoarthritis usually affects large weight–bearing joints such as the hip or knee, it is not uncommon in the hand.

Heberden's nodes

Clinical features
Present as small bony lumps at the terminal interphalangeal joints of the fingers (Fig. 118) and is more common in women.

Associated with formation of osteophytes (Fig. 119), the nodes may commence with redness and pain around the joint which usually settles after a few months.

Management
Pain and stiffness usually respond to analgesics.

Surgical fusion may be necessary in the occasional patient in whom pain is severe.

Mucous cyst

Clinical features
A cystic swelling arising from the dorsum of an osteoarthritic terminal interphalangeal joint (Fig. 120). Histologically the same as a ganglion (p. 65).

The cyst arises from one side of the extensor tendon and typically lies between the joint line and the nail fold. Mucous cysts within the nail fold can produce a longitudinal groove on the nail.

Occasionally the cyst becomes infected and may drain synovial fluid.

Management
Treatment is by aspiration. Surgical excision is an alternative but recurrence and skin breakdown are not uncommon complications.

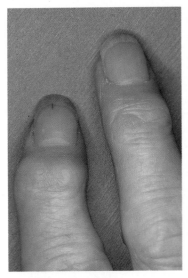
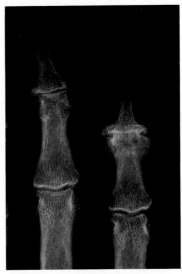

Fig. 118 Heberden's nodes.

Fig. 119 X-ray of Heberden's nodes.

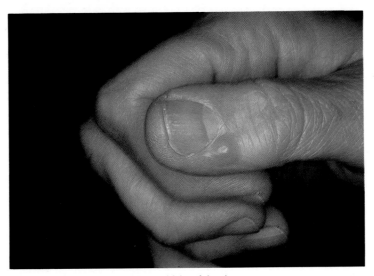

Fig. 120 Mucous cyst of interphalangeal joint of thumb.

Trapeziometacarpal joint of thumb

This is a common site for primary arthritis, particularly in middle-aged women.

Clinical features

Not always symptomatic it may cause local discomfort at the base of the thumb, especially when gripping or twisting off lids. In advanced cases a characteristic flexion–adduction deformity of the thumb metacarpal bone develops and is usually associated with compensatory hyperextension of the metacarpophalangeal joint (Fig. 121).

Radiological features

The earliest sign is narrowing of the joint space due to loss of articular cartilage. Later features include subluxation of the joint, sclerosis of bone adjacent to the joint and formation of osteophytes (Fig. 122).

Management

Treatment is with analgesia and support splint. Surgery is reserved for those who have significant disability due to pain that has not been relieved by conservative treatment. Various operations are used, including metacarpal osteotomy, excision of the trapezium (with or without prosthetic replacement) and total joint replacement.

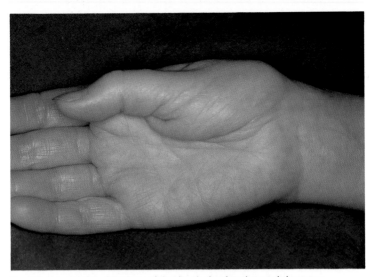

Fig. 121 Osteoarthritis of the base of the thumb showing characteristic posture.

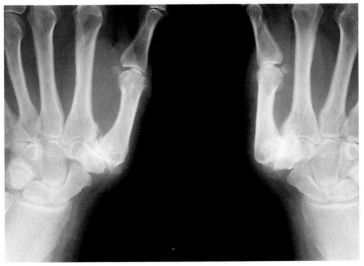

Fig. 122 Osteoarthritis affecting the trapeziopmetacarpal joints.

18 / **Other arthropathies**

Gout

A metabolic disorder in which there is deposition of monosodium urate in the periarticular tissues.

Aetiology Hyperuricaemia may be primary, in which case there is often a family history, or secondary to disorders such as polycythaemia, leukaemias or treatment with drugs, such as some diuretics.

Clinical features Middle–aged or elderly most often affected with sudden onset of swelling, redness and severe pain.

Gout usually affects a single joint, most often the first metatarsophalangeal joint or the knee, but a distal interphalangeal joint is occasionally involved (Fig. 123). The condition may then be misdiagnosed as paronychia (p. 55).

Investigations Serum urate level is usually raised in the acute attack but may be normal in chronic gout. X-ray may show joint destruction and swelling (Fig. 124).

Management Acute attack is controlled by anti–inflammatory drugs. Long-term treatment with a uricosuric agent is required to prevent recurrence.

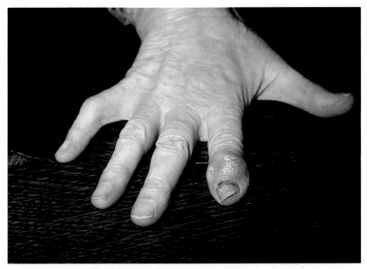

Fig. 123 Acute gout affecting the distal interphalangeal joint.

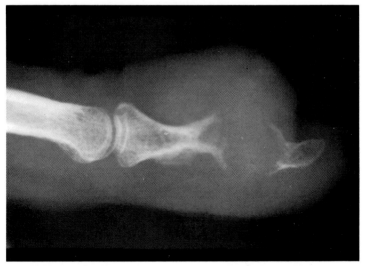

Fig. 124 X–ray of gouty joint.

Psoriasis

A common, chronic skin disorder characterized by raised, red, scaly patches of varying size. It may be associated with nail changes and damage to small joints in the hand. Aetiology is unknown.

Clinical features

The typical feature in the hand is pitting of the nails (Fig. 125), which sometimes occurs in the absence of the typical skin lesions.

Psoriatic arthropathy affects the small joints of the hand and occurs in up to 10% of those affected by psoriasis. The skin changes may be minor even when the arthropathy is severe but it is rare for joint changes to precede skin manifestations.

The joint changes are similar to those seen in rheumatoid arthritis but the metacarpophalangeal joints are less often affected. Occasionally there is marked destruction and severe deformity that may be sudden in onset and rapidly progressive (Fig. 126).

Management

Nail pitting may improve if the skin responds to dermatological treatment but the arthropathy is unaffected. Joint disease is treated with anti-inflammatory drugs. Surgical fusion of unstable joints may be necessary if destruction is severe.

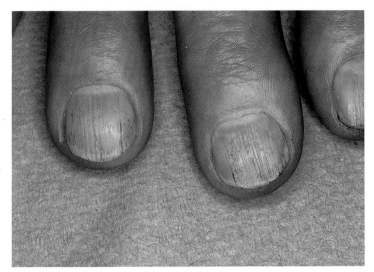

Fig. 125 Nail pitting in psoriasis.

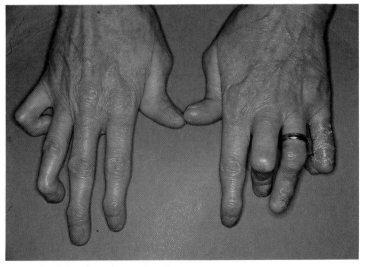

Fig. 126 Psoriatic arthropathy.

19 / Carpal tunnel syndrome

A disorder in which there is compression of the median nerve in the carpal tunnel beneath the flexor retinaculum at the wrist.

Incidence Carpal tunnel syndrome is very common with maximum incidence in middle-aged women.

Aetiology Frequently idiopathic but may be associated with rheumatoid arthritis, hypothyroidism, fluid retention during pregnancy or anatomical anomalies or tumours in the carpal tunnel.

Clinical features Typically the patient is woken during the night by pain that is often described as 'burning' or 'bursting'. The pain may not be confined to the distribution of the median nerve (p. 25). The discomfort is relieved by some activity such as shaking the hand, running cold water over it or getting up and moving about. The hand may feel heavy and numb in the morning.

On examination there is often no abnormality. Wasting of the thenar muscles (Fig. 127) is a very late feature. Unforced flexion of the wrist for about a minute precipitates the symptoms in about 75% of patients (Phalen's test, Fig. 128).

Slowing of conduction in the median nerve can be shown by electrophysiological testing but this is not necessary to make the diagnosis if the typical history is given.

Management **Conservative**: by splinting the wrist, diuretic drugs or injection of hydrocortisone into the carpal tunnel.
Surgical: decompression of the carpal tunnel by division of the flexor retinaculum.

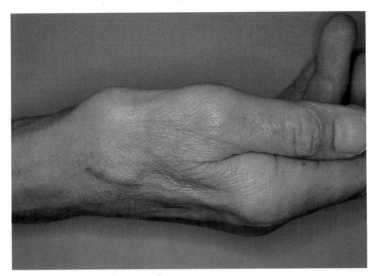

Fig. 127 Wasting of the thenar muscles.

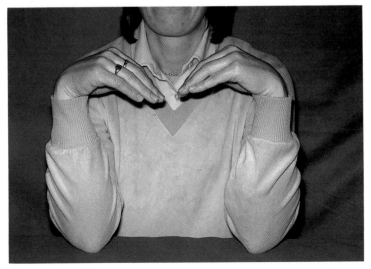

Fig. 128 Phalen's test.

20 / Stenosing tenosynovitis

De Quervain's tenosynovitis

An inflammatory, constricting synovitis of the first dorsal compartment of the wrist through which run the tendons of extensor pollicis brevis and abductor pollicis longus. Aetiology is uncertain.

Clinical features
De Quervain's tenosynovitis commonly affects middle-aged women. Presents as pain at the radial styloid process, aggravated by gripping when the wrist is ulnar deviated; this may cause heavy objects such as teapots to be dropped. The thickened sheath may be visible and palpable. Passive flexion of the thumb with the wrist ulnar deviated will reproduce the pain at the site (Finkelstein's test, Fig. 129).

Management
Conservative: splintage or injection of hydrocortisone into the affected compartment.
Surgical: decompression of the compartment. Care must be taken to avoid damage to the terminal branches of the radial nerve.

Trigger finger

A common condition in which a finger or thumb sticks in the flexed position (Fig. 130) due to narrowing of the proximal pulley of the flexor sheath or enlargement of the tendon. Common in rheumatoid arthritis.

Management
Conservative: hydrocortisone injection into the sheath.
Surgical: release of the proximal sheath.

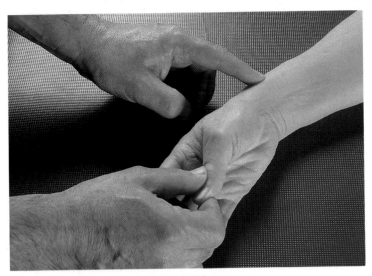

Fig. 129 De Quervain's tenosynovitis. Finkelstein's test.

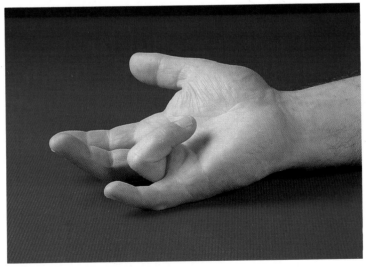

Fig. 130 Trigger finger. The typical position of flexion.

21 / Circulatory disorders

Scleroderma

A collagen disorder of unknown aetiology, characterized by sclerosis of the skin and alimentary tract, heart and lungs.

Pathology Fibrosis of affected structures associated with obliterative vascular changes.

Clinical features Scleroderma, which affects women much more often than men, may be preceded by Raynaud's disease, a painful condition affecting young women in which the fingers show abnormal vasoconstriction in response to cold.

Scleroderma affecting the hands (sclerodactyly) results in vasomotor disturbances, thickening and hardening of the skin, trophic changes (Fig. 131) and nodules of subcutaneous calcification (Fig. 132).

Management Symptomatic. Surgical removal of calcified nodules is sometimes necessary.

Acrocyanosis

Persistent cyanosis in the hands of young women without evidence of vascular disease (Fig. 133).

Aetiology Unknown. Sometimes familial.

Clinical features Worse in cold weather but painless and not associated with trophic changes.

Management Reassurance. Keep hands warm.

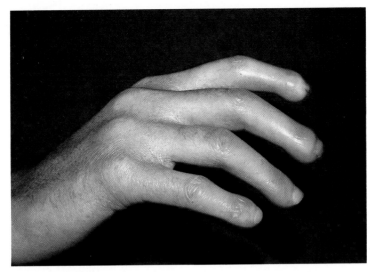

Fig. 131 Scleroderma.

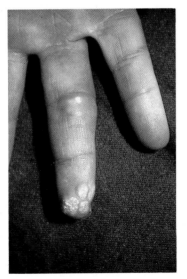

Fig. 132 Calcified nodules in scleroderma.

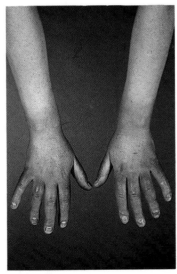

Fig. 133 Acrocyanosis.

22 / Nail disorders

See also glomus tumour (p. 69), malignant melanoma
(p. 73) and psoriasis (p. 93).

Splinter haemorrhages

Clinical features   Seen as small red streaks beneath the nail, with·
their long axes parallel to that of the nail (Fig. 134).

Causes   Classically they are associated with subacute bacterial
endocarditis, but they may also occur in minor
trauma, rheumatoid arthritis, psoriasis, dermatitis,
fungal infections and mitral stenosis.

Fungal infections

Common infection, especially in those whose hands
are often in water. Fungi can be demonstrated on
specially prepared nail clippings. *Trichophyton rubrum*
is the fungus most often isolated.

Clinical features   Affected nails become thickened, cracked and
discoloured (Fig. 135). Part of the nail may break
away.

Management   Avoidance of prolonged immersion and trauma helps.
Local antifungal agents may not be effective because
the infection is deep in the nail and its bed. Systemic
agents such as griseofulvin are effective but treatment
may have to be prolonged.

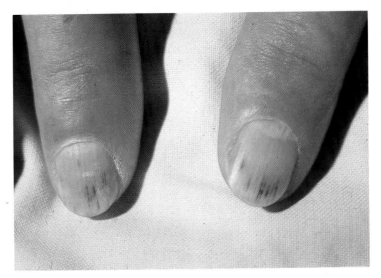

Fig. 134 Splinter haemorrhages.

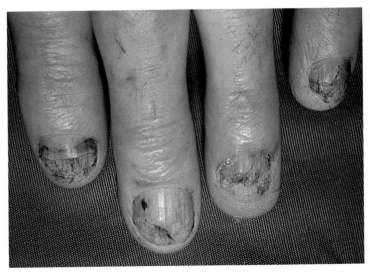

Fig. 135 Fungal infection.

Beau's lines

Clinical features   Seen as a depression across the surface of all nails (Fig. 136). In severe cases the nails may be shed.

Causes   The lines are the result of severe illnesses during which nail growth ceases. The nail changes are seen some weeks later when nail growth has recommenced. Beau's lines are typically seen after coronary thrombosis, severe chest infection, major trauma and, in children, measles.

Clubbing

Clinical features   There is loss of the normal angle between the nail and nail fold (Fig. 137) affecting all the nails.

Causes   The mechanism is uncertain but clubbing is possibly caused by increased blood flow and soft tissue proliferation in the terminal phalanges. Clubbing typically occurs in lung and heart disease associated with cyanosis. It may also be seen in thyroid disease, biliary cirrhosis and bowel disorders such as sprue and ulcerative colitis. Occasionally it is idiopathic and familial.

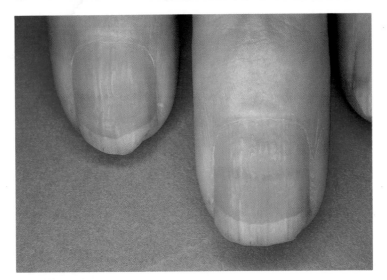

Fig. 136 Beau's lines.

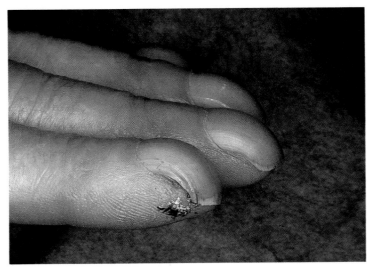

Fig. 137 Clubbing.

Index

Index